Rice Diet Handbook for Beginners:

Detailed Guide on How to Use Rice Diet to Lose Weight; Its Dos & Don'ts; Its Gains & Drawbacks; One(1) Week Rice Diet Plan & Lots More

By

Doctor Peter L. Turnbull

Copyright@2020

TABLE OF CONTENTS

CHAPTER ONE

INTRODUCTION

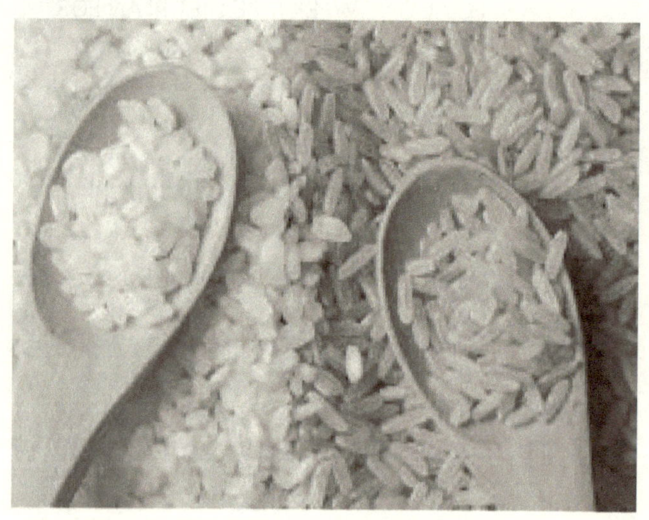

The rice diet is a high-intricate carb, low-fat, and low-sodium diet. It was initially evolved by Walter Kepmner, MD, a Duke University doctor in 1939. It recaptured prominence in 2006 after Kitty Gurkin Rosati, an enlisted dietician who represents considerable authority in the avoidance of heftiness, coronary illness, and other interminable infections

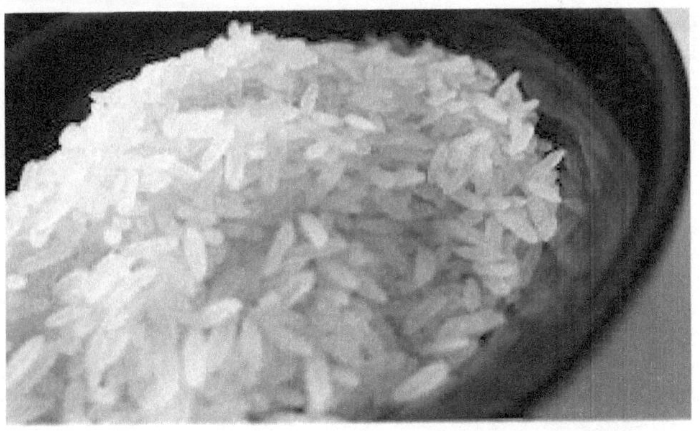

Rice as a piece of an eating routine

Each diet and every supper has a base. In the event that you are vegetarian, your dinners are presumably founded on grains, vegetables, and natural products. In the event that you follow an even eating routine, you may have potatoes, pasta, noodles, or rice as your base. Rice is generally utilized as a base in Asian nations and is additionally the primary part of the rice diet. The individuals who live in the previously mentioned Asian nations, for example, China, South Korea, and Japan are generally thin.

Indeed, even the insights show that these nations have an amazingly low level of individuals who are overweight or fat. It's no big surprise why the rice diet continues increasing more consideration. In any case, is eating rice actually the way to weight reduction and a fit body? To see if or not the rice diet will make you shed pounds, you have to comprehend the principle rules of this eating routine, and what are its advantages and drawbacks.

The idea of the rice diet

In spite of the fact that the rice diet has a long history of utilization, it is very well known these days, and with time acquires and more supporters. Its underlying essential use was to assist you with improving heart and kidney wellbeing and battle corpulence, yet as of now it is likewise broadly utilized for its weight reduction and detox impacts. It is a low-fat, low-sodium, low-protein, and low-calorie diet, which requires customary exercise and reflection. The everyday caloric breaking point in the primary period of the rice diet is 800 calories, which is practically nothing, taking into account that you ought to likewise consistently work out. After this stage, you are to expand the measure of devoured day by day calories to 1,000-1,200, and this number must continue as before until you arrive at your objective weight. Being profoundly prohibitive, it has the accompanying guidelines:

How the rice diet functions

Here, the eating routine works by concentrating on restricting salt and nourishments high in sodium. This will help your body de-swell and shed abundance water weight. In mix with eating low-sodium nourishments, the eating routine likewise restrains soaked fats.

Rather, it utilizes high-fiber nourishments to top you off and carbs like natural product, vegetables, grains, and beans, as the primary wellspring of sustenance. It additionally restricts practically all dairy from your eating routine.

The rice diet plan additionally follows a calorie stipend in case you're hoping to get in shape. At first, it suggests beginning at a lower calorie level and afterward developing to around 1,200 to 1,500 calories for every day in case you're not working out.

In the event that you follow the eating routine arrangement introduced in the book, you experience three expressions that train partition control and how to adjust food so you can have the opportunity to eat anything you desire with some restraint.

The see these rules rice diet plan that includes eating every day:

*1,000 calories

*500 to 1,000 mg of sodium

*22 g of fat

*5.5 g of soaked fat

*0 to 100 mg of cholesterol

What's more, as most top to bottom weight the board programs, the eating routine spotlights on way of life changes, such as keeping a food diary and investigating your relationship with food, your body, and self through contemplation, mindfulness, and diet.

Adequacy

As a rule, following any kind of supper plan that lessens calories and spotlights on vegetables and lean protein will be viable in helping you get thinner. Be that as it may, it's additionally imperative to ensure you're eating enough calories, as well. Contingent upon your digestion and exercise and movement levels, eating too barely any calories can really have the contrary impact on weight reduction. The next chapters

will explain all you need to know about rice diet
from a to z. Happy rice diet eating

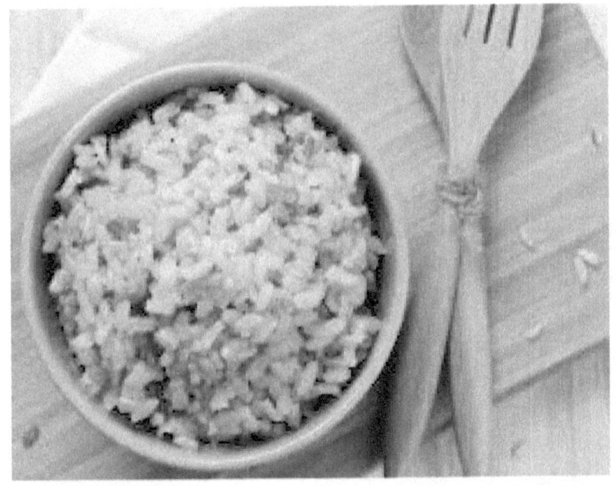

CHAPTER TWO

THE BENEFITS/GAINS OF RICE DIET, AND ITS DRAWBACKS YOU SHOULD KNOW

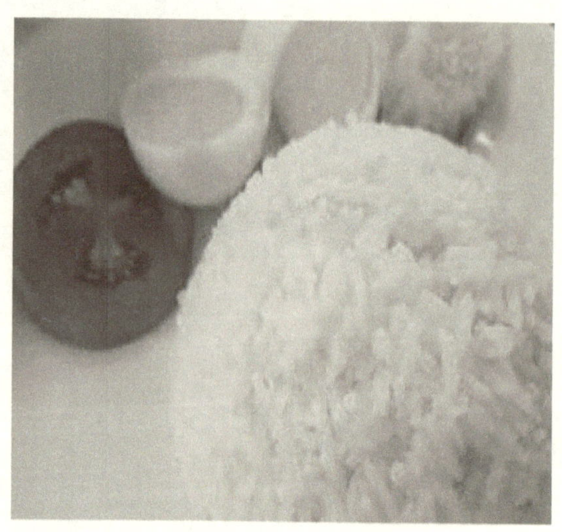

The advantages of the rice diet

The advantage of this eating regimen is that it can assist you with learning segment control and kick you off on eating all the more new foods grown from the ground. This kind of diet may likewise be exceptionally useful for somebody who has a heart condition that requires eating an eating routine low in sodium and fat.

Perhaps the greatest advantage of the rice diet is that it challenges that starches are a terrible thing. Such a large number of diets and wellbeing plans centre around eating low-carb food and dinners. They advance the possibility that carbs = evil. Yet, that is not simply false. Our bodies need starches to work effectively. Our minds need glucose to use as fuel. Carbs are companions, not enemies.

The way to eating carbs, obviously, is to eat the correct sort of carbs in the correct segment, which is the thing that this eating routine advances. The rice diet centres around complex starches like rice (nothing unexpected there), yams, or cereal, rather than basic carbs like treats and cake.

One lady who followed the eating routine composed a survey on Amazon. She noticed that for her, low-carb techniques just didn't work for her to get in shape. Each body is unique, and a few people may not react well to removing certain nutrition classes like carbs.

Definitely removing carbs can prompt weakness, cerebrum mist, and yearning — yet this eating regimen forestalls these side effects by keeping your body filled with complex carbs. Likewise, this eating regimen supports heaps of vegetables, which are viewed as incredible, supplement thick sugars.

Would it be a good idea for you to eat earthy colored rice or white rice?

You can eat either white or earthy colored rice on the eating regimen — giving the rice has no additional salt or fat. The first rice diet calls for utilizing white rice. At that point, it was simpler to make and more available.

Be that as it may, earthy colored rice is better known and open today. It's likewise not handled and is an entire grain with more fiber and supplement an incentive than white rice. In case you're focusing on eating totally natural nourishments, you might need to think about earthy colored rice.

More Explanation on The Advantages Of The Rice Diet

The rice diet has various advantages that may: improve your wellbeing, assist you with thinning down, and actualize some positive propensities into your everyday practice. They advantages are as follows:

1. Weight reduction

The way to effective weight reduction is the decrease of expended calories and an expansion in the measure of calories consumed. As the rice diet is exceptionally constraining regarding caloric admission and requires expanded standard physical action, you ought to have the option to shed the essential number of pounds to arrive at your objective weight and look after it. A Japanese report indicated that utilization of rice rather than bread for breakfast before practicing diminishes the opportunity of fat kept, implying that you won't just decrease the water weight, however will likewise dissolve away undesirable fat.

2. Improved kidney wellbeing

The rice diet is a low-sodium diet. Diminished sodium admission can keep your body from putting away water weight, yet what is more significant – battle or forestall kidney ailment. As one of the primary duties of your kidneys is to keep up a sound equalization of water, salts, and minerals, expanded utilization of sodium squeezes your kidneys, after some time causing the event of kidney maladies. To forestall this you ought to lessen the measure of salt that you eat, and that is the thing that the rice diet offers to you.

3. Lower pulse

Studies show that expanded sodium admission may prompt worse hypertension. Controlling the utilization of sodium through one's eating regimen has consistently been one of the best approaches to deal with that condition. In the event that you are not new to the universe of diets, you may have seen that the rice diet is to some degree like the DASH diet which is centred around battling hypertension. The primary concern these weight control plans share for all intents and purpose is the low sodium admission which is attached to all the more likely control of pulse.

Drawbacks of the rice diet

Great deals of weight reduction eats less carbs have certain drawbacks, and the rice diet isn't a special case. Here are a portion of the primary negative parts of this nourishment plan:

1. May prompt lacks

The constrained assortment of nourishments in this dietary arrangement may cause certain irregular characteristics in your body on the off chance that you tail it for a significant stretch of time. The diminished utilization of protein could cause loss of bulk. In the event that you don't take any enhancements while adhering to the rice diet, you may turn into a survivor of supplement inadequacy.

2. Hard to adhere to

As you definitely know, the rice diet is exceptionally constraining. That is the reason adhering to its arrangement for an extensive stretch of time might be troublesome and in any event, depleting, particularly when going to get-togethers or on the off chance that you are accustomed to eating out.

3. Not suggested for a drawn out use

In spite of the fact that the rice diet is staggeringly viable as a transient weight reduction, tailing it for quite a while may not be best for certain individuals. As it is extremely prohibitive and cuts the calorie and protein admission, the constrained sum may not be sufficient for certain individuals, over the long haul making hurt their health. On the off chance that you need to begin following this eating regimen, if it's not too much trouble examine every one of its angles with your primary care physician, choose whether it is ok for you and in what direction it is better for you to consolidate this eating routine or a portion of its standards into your daily schedule.

CHAPTER THREE

WHAT TO CONSUME ON A RICE DIET AS WELL AS TEST RICE DIET PLAN/RECIPES

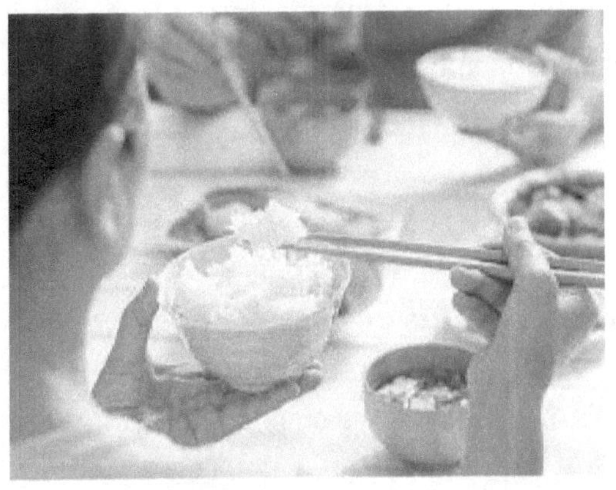

What to consume on the rice diet?

It has just been referenced that this eating regimen restricts the utilization of a great deal of nourishments, controlling you to expend solid carbs. Your suppers in this eating regimen may incorporate high-fiber foods grown from the ground, and grains, which are viewed as the fundamental segments of the eating routine. You can likewise eat natural, or negligibly handled beans. Basic nourishment for this eating regimen is low-or no-fat dairy items, for example, milk yogurt or curds. During the later stages, you are permitted to incorporate lean meats and fish into your dinner plan. As a rule, this eating regimen is low in nutrient/vitamin D and calcium and requires utilization of enhancements.

Dietary benefits of rice

As it's obvious from the name of the eating regimen, one of its primary fixings is rice and this is the reason you should know its dietary benefit. The two most famous gatherings of rice are white and earthy colored. White rice is an incredible wellspring of solid carbs, in actuality starches make up around 80% of its complete dry weight. Rice will in general assimilate a great deal of water while being cooked. In cooked structure 70% of its weight is comprised of water

Test rice diet plans

French toast

This formula can even be made early and warmed for occupied mornings.

Fixings:

*1 cup non-dairy milk

*1/2 cup squeezed orange

*2 tbsp. flour

*1 tbsp. sugar

*1 tbsp. healthful yeast

*1/2 tsp. cinnamon

*1/4 tsp. nutmeg

*6-8 cuts of bread

Bearings

Blend all fixings with the exception of the bread together. Dunk bread in the blend and warmth on a skillet.

Appetizing Rice

The rice diet wouldn't be finished without rice, isn't that so? This formula can be cooked and utilized for some servings consistently.

Fixings:

*1 cup earthy colored rice, cooked

*4 tbsp. onions, slashed

*2 tbsp. parsley, slashed

*2 cloves of garlic, minced

*1 tsp. paprika

Headings:

Warmth the garlic and onion with the rice, at that point sprinkle with the parsley and paprika while still warm.

CHAPTER FOUR

RICE MENU FOR YOU AND SOME THINGS TO AVOID

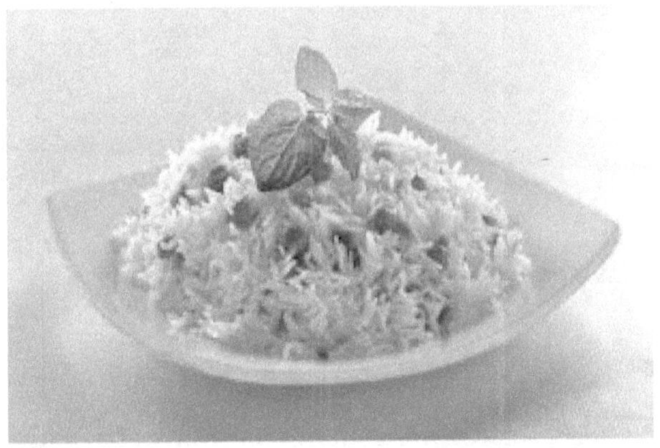

Rice diet menu

One cup of cooked white rice (205g) contains:

*Calories – 266 kcal

*Fats – 0.389 g

*Carbs – 58.9 g

*Protein – 4.84 g

*Water – 140 g

Earthy colored rice contains more fiber, fat, and protein than white rice. It is additionally more extravagant in manganese, phosphorus, magnesium, and niacin, and is viewed as somewhat more advantageous than the white. In this way, it is up to you which to pick. Other than rice, you may likewise eat bread or pasta, yet in addition in a limited quantity.

On the off chance that you've assembled up the mental fortitude to smash your weight reduction objective. Our application will assist you with rebuilding your propensities, remould your life and wrench up your wellness results!

What to stay away from?

As should be obvious, the rice diet is very constraining of nourishments and calories thus it might require clinical oversight. When following a rice diet, you ought to keep away from nourishments that are pungent, prepared, oily, and wealthy in fats. Liquor and desserts, including pastries and sweet beverages, are likewise not for you on the off chance that you adhere to this wholesome arrangement. You ought to likewise consider decreasing the size of your bits so as to arrive at the ideal outcome.

CHAPTER FIVE

A SPECIAL ONE WEEK RICE DIET PLAN FOR YOU

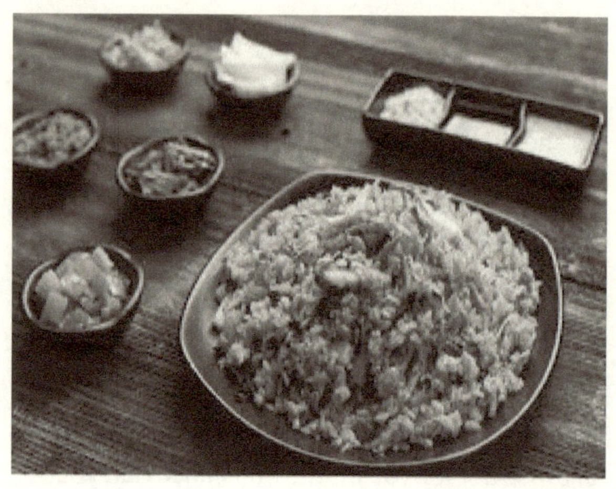

One Week Rice Diet Plan Plus Its Gains

Rice Diet

Rice diet is a solid eating regimen. Organic products, grains and high fiber vegetables make up the majority of the eating routine. Rice diet is low in fat and furthermore in salt. Day by day rice diet contains 800 calories for each day which is low. An eating regimen which is wealthy in vegetables, organic products, entire grains and low in sugar these are keep you from numerous medical issues like disease, heart issues, diabetes and hypertension. Your day by day dinner ought not the same as stage one. In stage two you can eat in one day of week fish, lean meat or eggs. This stage can assist you with controlling your weight. Stage three us likewise called look after stage, it is proposed to be your dietary arrangement for your up and coming life. In all stages you need to avoid salt or fat. Earthy colored rice which is less prepared and loaded up with supplements and fiber and solid than white rice as well as helps one to lose fats in your body and keep you sound. Earthy colored rice have nutrients, amino acids and minerals, it is that wellspring of dietary which help to battle with clogging. Rice diet is excellent for your body and gives you vitality, earthy colored rice is comprises of complex starch and conveyed vitality giving sugars gradually. Rice gives you about 21% of worldwide human per capita vitality and 15% capita protein. Rice protein positions is high in supplements among grains, it additionally gives minerals, nutrient and fiber. Minerals and nutrient increment the capacity and metabolic action of all your body organs and furthermore increment vitality levels. Rice diet is likewise useful for your heart wellbeing. Grain oil which is produced using rice it contain ground-breaking cancer prevention agents that make spare your heart from numerous different issues.

Rice diet plan is solid in light of the fact that

*It purifies the entire body

*It is satisfying

*It is low in calorie

*It is delightful

7 days rice diet plan

Monday:

Breakfast: eat ½ cup of earthy colored rice, 1 apples and 1 cup of green tea

Lunch: ½ cup of earthy colored rice, vegetable soup with serving of mixed greens

Supper: earthy colored rice

Tuesday:

Breakfast: eat any organic product don't eat bananas or grapes or earthy colored rice

Lunch: veggies, bubbled fish or vegetable soup

Supper: virgin coconut oil or earthy colored rice with little margarine

Wednesday:

Breakfast: one apple, earthy colored rice

Lunch: cucumber serving of mixed greens, vegetable soup

Supper: enormous plate of mixed greens and heated mushroom

Thursday:

Breakfast: plain yogurt with earthy colored rice

Lunch: serving of mixed greens, vegetables soup
and 2 oz. of lean meat

Supper: earthy colored rice with vegetables

Friday:

Breakfast: earthy colored rice and on organic
product

Lunch: fish, serving of mixed greens, vegetable
soup, earthy colored rice

Supper: earthy colored rice and serving of mixed greens

Saturday:

Breakfast: a few pecans, one apples and earthy colored rice

Lunch: serving of mixed greens, lean meat, steamed veggies vegetables soup and earthy colored rice

Supper: virgin coconut oil or earthy colored rice with little margarine

Sunday:

Breakfast: one foods grown from the ground rice

Lunch: fish, earthy colored rice, beans and
vegetable soup

Supper: serving of mixed greens with olives,
earthy colored rice and enormous plate of mixed
greens.

CHAPTER SIX

FURTHER IDEAS ABOUT RICE DIET, AND SOME VITAL FACTS

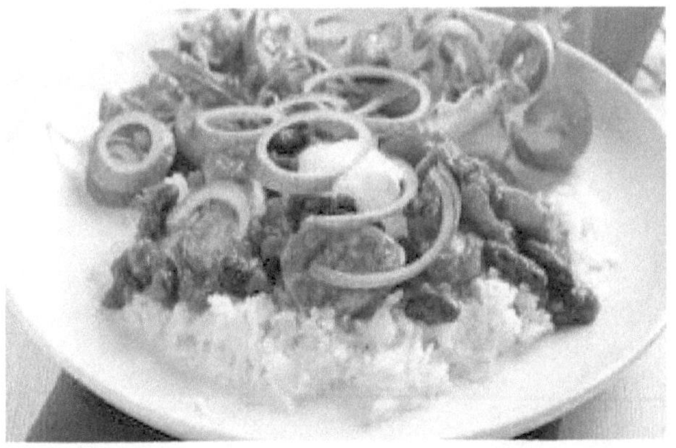

Rice diet dinner thoughts for you

Utilizing rice as a dinner base has a long history, and there are a variety of dishes that incorporate this fixing and might be consolidated into the rice diet feast plan. Evaluating the accompanying dishes may add some flavour to your eating routine, and zest up your dietary daily practice:

*Vegetable and rice pilaf

*Sautéed veggies with rice

*Mushroom risotto

*Sushi burrito

*Steamed salmon and vegetable rice bowl

*Mango clingy rice

*Omurice (omelet on rice)

*Chicken Spinach Artichoke Rice Casserole

*Plates of mixed greens with rice

*Rice puddings

*Chicken and rice diet

Rice diet plan test

As you definitely know, the rice diet comprises of three stages. The motivation behind the principal stage is to detox your body and purge you from the abundance measure of sodium, refined carbs, and unfortunate fats. The subsequent stage focuses on wellbeing improvement and weight reduction, so it goes on until you arrive at your ideal weight. What's more, the third stage is intended to assist you with executing smart dieting propensities and keep up your outcomes. Each stage has its caloric and food limitations thus, unique feast plans. Here is an example rice diet plan for each stage:

Stage 1 – 800 calories

Breakfast: some oats with orange and chia seeds, some unsweetened green tea.

Lunch: A cup of rice, half of a cup of pan-seared vegetables.

Tidbit: A cup of nonfat yogurt with berries.

Supper: Grilled vegetables and mushroom rice, some unsweetened natural tea.

Rice diet

Stage 2 – 1,000 calories

Breakfast: One cut of toast, half of an avocado, and a large portion of some curds, some unsweetened green tea.

Lunch: A cup of rice, a large portion of a cup of pan-seared vegetables, half of a flame broiled chicken bosom.

Tidbit: Cups of organic product blend (apples, oranges, bananas, pears).

Supper: Vegetable and fish sushi, some unsweetened home grown tea.

Stage 3 – 1,200 calories

Breakfast: some vegetable quinoa, some unsweetened green tea.

Lunch: A cup of rice, a large portion of a cup of pan-seared vegetables, a medium-sized heated fish.

Tidbit: A cup of unsweetened yogurt with dried foods grown from the ground.

Supper: Chicken bosom and mushroom risotto, some unsweetened home grown tea.

Different kinds of rice abstains from food

There are various kinds of rice abstains from food, each with its standards, limitations, and objectives. Despite the fact that they all have rice in their names, they despite everything have distinctive rice diet menus. This is the reason you ought to painstakingly pick which intend to follow, as it might cause the contrary impact of what you anticipate.

The most well-known kinds of the rice eats less carbs are chicken and rice diet, rice and beans diet, and an earthy colored rice diet. They are for the most part dependent on rice, which if over devoured may have certain negative results. Studies show that expanded utilization of rice may prompt a higher danger of type 2 diabetes.

There is research anyway that has indicated that this subject requires further examination and it is too soon to broadcast its destructive impact dependent on the proof that has been introduced up until now.

Vital Facts You Should Know

Again, as was explained in chapter two, the restricted assortment of nourishments in this dietary arrangement may cause certain awkward nature in your body on the off chance that you tail it for an extensive stretch of time. The diminished utilization of protein could cause loss of bulk. On the off chance that you don't take any enhancements while adhering to the rice diet, you may turn into a survivor of supplement lack.

As you definitely know, the rice diet is exceptionally restricting. That is the reason adhering to its arrangement for a significant stretch of time might be extremely troublesome and in any event, debilitating, particularly when going to get-togethers or in the event that you are accustomed to eating out.

CHAPTER SEVEN

A FINAL WORD FOR YOU

In case you're keen on attempting the rice diet strategy, talk with your primary care physician before rolling out any radical improvements to your eating routine, particularly in the event that you have any ailments that influence your sodium levels.

Remember that there's nothing of the sort as a "diet" for weight reduction. Rather, fuse way of life changes that can assist you with keeping up a sound weight.

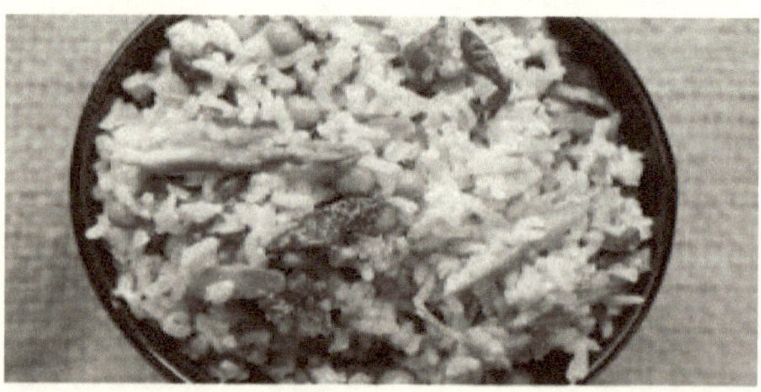

The rice diet was first made to improve your wellbeing by battling corpulence and cardiovascular infections, advancing kidney wellbeing, and bringing down circulatory strain. Because of its adequacy for weight reduction, individuals use it to thin down and detox the body. The rice diet has an extraordinary number of limitations, constraining your food admission to products of the soil, grains, a few beans and low-or non-fat dairy in the main stage, and permitting some lean meats and fish in the second.

While utilizing standard exercises, it requires a serious modest number of calories thus this isn't sufficient for certain individuals. In spite of the fact that this wholesome arrangement has certain medical advantages, including weight reduction, improved kidney wellbeing, and others, it despite everything has its drawbacks, which may make it troublesome and unsafe for specific individuals to follow this arrangement for a significant stretch of time. As this eating regimen was made for restorative purposes, and is very exacting, it might require clinical management. Before bringing this eating routine into your everyday routine, if you don't mind counsel a pro.

THE END